BEGINNER'S GUIDE TO THE BENEFITS OF MAGNESIUM

Reduces Anxiety; Eases Depression; Enhances Sleep; Relieves Muscle Cramps; Reduces Symptoms of PMS and Menopause; Detoxifies the Body; Builds Stronger Bones

Copyright © 2022 by Darlene Brieno

All rights reserved. No part of this publication may be reproduced, stored or transmitted in any form or by any means, electronic, mechanical, photocopying, recording, scanning, or otherwise without written permission from the publisher. It is illegal to copy this book, post it to a website, or distribute it by any other means without permission.

Darlene Brieno asserts the moral right to be identified as the author of this work.

Darlene Brieno has no responsibility for the persistence or accuracy of URLs for external or third-party Internet Websites referred to in this publication and does not guarantee that any content on such Websites is, or will remain, accurate or appropriate.

Designations used by companies to distinguish their products are often claimed as trademarks. All brand names and product names used in this book and on its cover are trade names, service marks, trademarks and registered trademarks of their respective owners. The publishers and the book are not associated with any product or vendor mentioned in this book. None of the companies referenced within the book have endorsed the book.

First edition

This book was professionally typeset on Reedsy.
Find out more at reedsy.com

Contents

Acknowledgement		iv
1	Magnesium Basics	1
2	Factors that Contribute to Magnesium Deficiency	4
3	What are Common Symptoms and Conditions Associated with...	7
4	How is Magnesium Deficiency Diagnosed?	10
5	Are you suffering from magnesium deficiency?	12
6	How is Magnesium Deficiency Treated?	15
7	What does magnesium deficiency look like?	18
8	Three Conditions Caused by a Magnesium Deficiency That may...	21
9	Depression	24
10	Insomnia	29
11	Conclusion	36
12	Resources	37

Acknowledgement

1

Magnesium Basics

DISCLAIMER

The information presented is the author's opinion and does not constitute any health or medical advice. The content of this book is for informational purposes only and is not intended to diagnose, treat, cure, or prevent any condition or disease. In no manner should this book or any of the information in this book be used as a substitute for diagnosis or treatment by a qualified medical or dental healthcare professional

Why is Magnesium Important?

I've written this book to help educate on the importance of magnesium and why you should learn about this mineral. What follows may be a little technical, but stick with it. This information will help you identify deficiency symptoms you may be experiencing and then learn what to do about it.

Magnesium is a metallic ion that is used in more than 300 enzyme systems. These systems regulate distinct biochemical reactions in the body, including protein synthesis, muscle and nerve function, blood glucose control, and blood pressure regulation. Magnesium is also necessary for energy, DNA, and RNA production, and it is part of the calcium and potassium ion transport system across cell membranes. This is important for nerve impulse conduction, muscle contraction and normal heart rhythm.

It is a mineral that is used by every organ of the body. This mineral plays an integral role in the heart, the muscles and kidneys. It is also one of the minerals that contributes to bone structure and is the fourth most abundant cation in the body.

What makes Magnesium so Essential to life?

This magical mineral has two super-powers. One is the ability to form chelates. In simple terms, a chelate is an organic compound that is bonded to a metal atom. This super-power is very important in metabolism and energy production. The second super-power is its ability to compete with calcium at binding sites on proteins and membranes. Without this super-power, proteins used in metabolism could not be created and organ systems that depend on magnesium would fail.

When magnesium competes with calcium for membrane binding sites, it works to maintain calcium levels in the correct proportion inside and outside of our cells. Calcium constricts smooth muscle and magnesium dilates smooth muscle. This helps explain how magnesium can decrease high blood pressure through the relaxation of the smooth muscles of the blood vessels. Magnesium ensures that the electrical properties of our cell membranes are kept in balance as it works in conjunction with potassium and calcium. Knowing this, we can see why the nervous system is affected by magnesium deficiency. If our electrical processes are off balance, our nervous system is not going to function at peak performance.

Admittedly, this is a very simplistic explanation of a very complicated topic. However, I think we all get the message that magnesium is essential to life. Educating yourself on this topic could be life changing if you are currently in a deficient state.

2

Factors that Contribute to Magnesium Deficiency

Because it is used in many functions of the body, especially metabolism, deficiency symptoms vary according to the body function that is affected. If magnesium levels drop too low, seizures could occur or the heart could go into a fatal arrhythmia. Magnesium balance is maintained by the kidneys where magnesium reabsorption occurs.

What are common causes of low magnesium levels?

There are various causes that contribute to low magnesium levels. Certain disease conditions put you at higher risk of becoming deficient. The List below is not all inclusive but it will give you a better understanding as to what may have caused your magnesium deficiency.

- Type 2 Diabetes
- Alcohol dependence
- Chronic diarrhea

FACTORS THAT CONTRIBUTE TO MAGNESIUM DEFICIENCY

- Long-term vomiting
- Excessive urination. This may be caused by caffeine due to its diuretic effect on the body
- Hypoaldosteronism, an adrenal gland condition that causes too much of the hormone aldosterone to be released into the blood
- Kidney problems
- Fluoride and fluorine bind with magnesium so that it becomes unavailable to the body. These chemicals may be found in the water, dental procedures, toothpaste and some medications
- Chlorine and calcium in the water will cause magnesium deficiency
- Long term use of diuretics (water pills)
- Malabsorption syndromes, such as Celiac disease, Crohn's disease, inflammatory bowel disease and others
- Malnutrition can occur due to eating a poor diet, starvation, eating disorders, digestive problems and any medical condition that makes it difficult for a person to eat
- Medicines including cisplatin, cyclosporine, diuretics, proton pump inhibitors, and aminoglycoside antibiotics. There are many other medications, speak to your pharmacist to learn more about your prescribed medications
- Pancreatitis (swelling and inflammation of the pancreas)
- Excessive sweating such as occurs with exercise, working in hot temperatures, during use of a sauna and other sweat inducing activities
- Eating food that is deficient in magnesium. This results with land overuse. The land itself becomes magnesium deficient and therefore the produce grown on the land is deficient
- "Hungry bone syndrome" after parathyroid or thyroid surgery
- Cooked food has lower levels of magnesium because some is destroyed during processing and cooking
- Gastric bypass surgery

- Low levels of potassium will cause an increased loss of magnesium through the urine
- Stress
- Tannin, a naturally occurring substance in tea, binds and removes minerals, including magnesium
- Some herbicides bind with magnesium making it unavailable to growing plants
- Highly process foods and foods high in sugar deplete magnesium during the digestive process. The liver requires 28 atoms of magnesium to process one molecule of glucose. Fructose requires 56 atoms of magnesium to process one molecule of glucose.
- Mercury amalgam dental fillings
- Taking calcium or zinc without taking magnesium

It's important to keep in mind that the symptoms listed above have many other causes. For example, stress or excessive caffeine could also cause involuntary muscle spasms. Medications may cause side effects that are similar or muscle spasms may be a symptom of a neuromuscular disease such as multiple sclerosis. However, if your symptoms are occurring due to a magnesium deficiency, you can reverse them simply by taking magnesium. It's a simple, inexpensive remedy.

3

What are Common Symptoms and Conditions Associated with Magnesium Deficiency?

When magnesium levels begin to drop below normal levels symptoms will develop. In some cases, deficiency may not be diagnosed because the obvious symptoms may not appear until magnesium levels become severely low.

Prolonged low magnesium levels are often associated with chronic diseases. These include diabetes, high blood pressure, heart disease, and osteoporosis. Magnesium has been used to treat asthma, heart attacks and pre-eclampsia, a condition that occurs to pregnant women. This seems to indicate that in some cases, magnesium deficiency is implicated in the disease process.

Since magnesium is used in many functions of the body, symptoms are variable and are dependent on the particular body function. For example, how are muscles affected by low magnesium levels? Common symptoms affecting the muscles and other body symptoms include:

- Muscle cramps or spasms in any muscle, including the heart. Do you have an irregular heart beat? Ask your physician to test your magnesium levels. Do your toes or calves cramp up? Magnesium deficiency may be the culprit.
- Abnormal eye movements or eye twitching.
- Headaches due to muscle tension and spasms
- Seizures or convulsions
- Teeth grinding and jaw pain if jaw muscles are tight due to deficiency
- Muscle weakness
- Back pain due to tense, tight muscles
- Abnormal heart rhythms
- Heart disease Fun fact: The left ventricle of the heart muscle has the highest concentration of magnesium as compared to any other muscle in the body. With magnesium deficiency, your heart muscle can experience abnormal heart rhythms
- Hyper-excitability or irritability
- High blood pressure can be caused by spasms of the smooth muscles that line the inside of the blood vessels
- Hypoglycemia is caused when too much insulin is released at one time causing the blood sugar levels to drop too low. Magnesium regulates insulin production and helps stabilize blood sugar levels
- Acid reflux (due to esophageal spasm, which can cause the esophageal sphincter to stay open)
- Fatigue
- Asthma
- Atherosclerosis and arthritis with calcium deposits. Magnesium works to dissolve calcium and to keep it soluble in the bloodstream and protects bone integrity by directing calcium to the bone.
- Constipation
- Bladder irritability caused by bladder muscle spasms

- Inflammation is caused when the inflammatory cascade is triggered by magnesium deficiency and calcium excess
- Depression
- Anxiety and panic attacks
- Osteoporosis
- Toxic body: Magnesium removes heavy metals from the body through the production of glutathione and the detox pathway in the liver. You are at risk of poisoning from mercury, aluminum and lead if you are deficient in magnesium as these heavy metals can build up in your body
- Sleep disorders can occur because of muscle tension and also because melatonin cannot be produced naturally in the body without sufficient magnesium.
- Kidney stones can develop with deficiency of magnesium and low levels of B6
- Nerve pain known as neuralgia and neuropathy occurs when the nerves suffer from sustained excitability due to magnesium deficiency. These manifest as numbness, prickling, skin sensitivity, tingling skin
- Confusion and dizziness
- Premenstrual syndrome
- Painful cramping during a woman's period
- Female infertility if caused by muscle spasms of the Fallopian tubes
- Premature contractions during pregnancy
- Preeclampsia and eclampsia in pregnancy
- Male infertility if magnesium and zinc are deficient. Normally both are present at healthy levels in semen

4

How is Magnesium Deficiency Diagnosed?

Magnesium deficiency is diagnosed using a blood test. If you are experiencing symptoms of magnesium deficiency, notify your physician and ask for a blood test to check your levels. Your physician may also suspect magnesium deficiency if you have abnormal calcium or potassium levels. Currently there is no easy test to measure magnesium levels. Serum magnesium and the magnesium tolerance test are the most widely used. Measurement of ionized magnesium provides more accurate results but is not widely available. This type of testing is available only through specialized labs. Per the National Institutes of Health (NIH), Office of Dietary Supplements,

"Assessing magnesium status is difficult because most magnesium is inside cells or in bone [3]. The most commonly used and readily available method for assessing magnesium status is measurement of serum magnesium concentration, even though serum levels have little correlation with total body magnesium levels or concentrations in specific tissues [6]. Other methods for assessing magnesium status include measuring magnesium concentrations in erythrocytes, saliva, and urine; measuring ionized magnesium concentrations in blood, plasma, or serum; and conducting a magnesium-loading (or "tolerance") test. No single method is considered satisfactory [7]. Some experts [4] but not others [3] consider the tolerance test (in which urinary magnesium is measured after parenteral infusion of a dose of magnesium) to be the best method to assess magnesium status in adults. To comprehensively evaluate magnesium status, both laboratory tests and a clinical assessment might be required [6]."

How can Magnesium Blood Levels be Normal and a Person still be Deficient?

Magnesium is so important to life that your body will leach it out of your bones in order to keep blood levels normal. If you have a history of heavy exercise or have worked in a job that causes you to sweat a lot, you are at risk for magnesium deficiency. You are losing magnesium through your skin while sweating. According to the NIH, your physician should take both your laboratory results and your symptoms into account when diagnosing magnesium deficiency. If you don't want to go through all the trouble of getting tested, ask your physician if you have health condition that would make it unsafe for you to take magnesium, for example, chronic kidney failure. Once you get the green light from your physician, take magnesium according to the instructions on the label or as prescribed by your physician. It may take a few weeks to a few months for you to experience the full benefit of this magical mineral. This will depend on how deficient you are. But stick with it. You won't be sorry.

5

Are you suffering from magnesium deficiency?

Before reading the next section, which discusses treatment options, take a moment and read over the list of symptoms and disease conditions that occur when the body is in a deficient state. Place a check mark next to each symptom or condition that you are currently suffering from. Be sure to write the date down as well. This is a great list to discuss with your physician on your next visit. Get the green light to take a magnesium supplement and begin eating foods that have high levels of magnesium per serving size. Once a month, recheck the list. Which symptoms are improving? By tracking your progress each month, you will be able to look back and see all the improvements in your health. If any symptom persists or gets worse at any time, see your physician.

Today's Date: _____

Place a Check mark Next to Each Symptom you are Currently Experiencing:

- Muscle cramps or spasms in any muscle, including the heart. Do you have an irregular heart beat? Ask your physician to test your magnesium levels. Do your toes or calves cramp up? Magnesium deficiency may be the culprit.
- Abnormal eye movements or eye twitching.
- Headaches due to muscle tension and spasms
- Seizures or convulsions
- Teeth grinding and jaw pain if jaw muscles are tight due to deficiency
- Muscle weakness
- Back pain due to tense, tight muscles
- Abnormal heart rhythms
- Heart disease Fun fact: The left ventricle of the heart muscle has the highest concentration of magnesium as compared to any other muscle in the body. With magnesium deficiency, your heart muscle can experience abnormal heart rhythms
- Hyperexcitability or irritability
- High blood pressure can be caused by spasms of the smooth muscles that line the inside of the blood vessels
- Hypoglycemia that is caused when too much insulin is released at one time causing the blood sugar levels to drop too much. Magnesium regulates insulin production
- Acid reflux (due to esophageal spasm, which can cause the esophageal sphincter to stay open)
- Fatigue
- Asthma
- Atherosclerosis and arthritis with calcium deposits. Magnesium works to dissolve calcium and to keep it soluble in the bloodstream and protects bone integrity by directing calcium to the bone.
- Constipation
- Bladder irritability caused by bladder muscle spasms

- Inflammation is caused when the inflammatory cascade is triggered by magnesium deficiency and calcium excess
- Depression
- Anxiety and panic attacks
- Osteoporosis
- Toxic body:Magnesium removes heavy metals from the body through the production of glutathione and the detox pathway in the liver.You are at risk of poisoning from mercury, aluminum and lead if you are deficient in magnesium as these heavy metals can build up in your body
- Sleep disorders can occur because of muscle tension and also because melatonin cannot be produced naturally in the body without sufficient magnesium.
- Kidney stones can develop with deficiency of magnesium and low levels of B6
- Nerve pain known as neuralgia and neuropathy occurs when the nerves suffer from sustained excitability due to magnesium deficiency. These manifest as numbness, prickling, skin sensitivity, tingling skin
- Confusion and dizziness
- Premenstrual syndrome
- Painful cramping during a woman's period
- Female infertility if caused by muscle spasms of the Fallopian tubes
- Premature contractions during pregnancy
- Preeclampsia and eclampsia in pregnancy
- Male infertility if magnesium and zinc are deficient. Normally both are present at healthy levels in semen
- Tooth decay due to imbalance of phosphorus and calcium in the saliva. This imbalance is caused by magnesium deficiency

6

How is Magnesium Deficiency Treated?

Depending on how mild or severe the magnesium deficiency is, it can be treated by:

- eating foods high in magnesium;
- taking magnesium supplements;
- Soaking in an Epsom salt bath or treating yourself to a Float Spa;
- Soaking your feet in an Epsom salt foot bath
- Rubbing magnesium oil on your skin;
- If you are severely deficient, your physician may opt to give you magnesium via intravenous infusion.
- Please remember, magnesium is an integral mineral, but more is NOT better. Work with your physician to determine dosage.

If you eat a poor diet, eat lots of sugary or process foods, or can't tolerate foods high in magnesium, work with your physician to discover the correct dose and form of magnesium supplement that works best for you. Some forms of magnesium are more difficult to absorb. Because of this they can cause diarrhea. I have found that magnesium glycinate and magnesium citrate are well tolerated by my body. Per the National Institutes of Health (NIH), Office of Dietary Supplements,

"Absorption of magnesium from different kinds of magnesium supplements varies. Forms of magnesium that dissolve well in liquid are more completely absorbed in the gut than less soluble forms [2,12]. Small studies have found that magnesium in the aspartate, citrate, lactate, and chloride forms is absorbed more completely and is more bioavailable than magnesium oxide and magnesium sulfate [12-16]."

Refer to Table 1 below for Recommended Dietary Allowances for Magnesium by age. These recommendations were published by the National Institutes of Health, Office of Dietary Supplements, Fact sheet for Health professionals.

Table 1: Recommended Dietary Allowances (RDAs) for Magnesium				
Age	Male	Female	Pregnancy	Lactation
Birth to 6 months	30 mg*	30mg*		
7 - 12 months	75 mg*	75 mg*		
1 - 3 years	80 mg	80 mg		
4 - 8 years	130 mg	130 mg		
9 - 13 years	240 mg	240 mg		
14 - 18 years	410 mg	360 mg	400 mg	360 mg
19 - 30 years	400 mg	310 mg	350 mg	310 mg
31 - 50 years	420 mg	320 mg	360 mg	320 mg
51+ years	420 mg	320 mg		

Foods High in Magnesium

In general, foods that are high in magnesium include green leafy vegetables such as spinach. Legumes, nuts, seeds and whole grains are also good sources of magnesium. Refer to Table 2 for a list of ten foods that are high in magnesium.

Table 2: Ten Foods High in Magnesium

Food	Serving Size	Magnesium
Brazil Nuts	1 ounce	107 mg
Black Beans	1 cup	120 mg
Pumpkin Seeds	1 ounce	150 mg
Cooked Spinach	1 cup	157 mg
Zucchini Squash	1 cup	20 mg
Chickpeas	1 cup	230 mg
Kale raw & chopped	1 cup	31 mg
Dark Chocolate	1 ounce	64 mg
Almonds	1 ounce	80 mg
Cashews	1 ounce	82 mg

7

What does magnesium deficiency look like?

A*Real Life Example:*

To answer this question, I thought it would be easiest to share my own experience to help you visualize how a deficiency can manifest. Your experience will be different, depending on how mild or severe your deficiency is.

Three years ago, I found myself sitting with my physician discussing magnesium supplementation because I was experiencing a constellation of symptoms. I was waking up at night with cramps in my calves and toes. My cramps were so painful, I had to jump out of bed and try to stamp them out. I was suffering from chronic pain in the muscles of my back, shoulders and neck area. Deep massage only helped temporarily. My right eye was twitching and I was experiencing heart palpitations. I was also having anxiety attacks, but at the time, I didn't know it was related to my magnesium deficiency.

When my physician reviewed my blood work, he noted that my calcium and potassium levels were low but my magnesium levels were normal.

Based on my symptoms and the calcium and potassium levels, my physician diagnosed mild magnesium deficiency. He advised that I take magnesium daily according to the labeling on the bottle.

It took nearly six months for all my symptoms to be resolved. My insomnia was the first symptom to be relieved. I began to sleep better and longer through the night. This was a bonus benefit. I hadn't realized the full impact of my insomnia until my sleep improved. I no longer became sleepy while driving or when I sat down to watch TV. Eventually my heart palpitations, leg cramps and eye twitch were gone. My back pain was the last to be resolved and if I fail to take my magnesium supplements for longer than a week, this symptom is the first to reappear. All my muscles relaxed after I started taking magnesium and the muscle aches, tension and pain in my back and shoulders is completely gone.

I have suffered from anxiety for most of my life. My father was an anxious person. My grandmother and all my uncles on my Dad's side also suffered from anxiety. I figured it was in my genetic make-up and I couldn't change it or make it better because genetic problems can't be fixed. Studies show that your genes may predispose you to certain medical conditions but it's your lifestyle and diet that "pull the trigger" so to speak. However, after taking magnesium for several months, I noticed that even my anxiety was diminished. In my case, it wasn't just my genes that were the problem. My body needed magnesium.

Anxiety occurs from multiple causes, but for me, one of the causes was magnesium deficiency. I no longer experience panic attacks. I remember a couple of times when I was driving I had to pull off to the side of the road and walk up and down the side of the road just to walk off the racing heart rate and the panic. My anxiety is now a low-grade condition. I'm mostly free of anxiety, but I can still work myself up. However, that's a different problem, unrelated to magnesium deficiency.

I've been taking magnesium supplements for the past three years. Sometimes I go to the Float Spa and soak for an hour in a magnesium pool. It's so relaxing. I also soak my feet in an Epsom salt foot bath a couple of times per week. I do this as part of my bedtime ritual because it makes me drowsy and I find it easier to fall asleep.

It's important that you select a type of magnesium that is easy to absorb. It is believed that the organic salt chelates such as magnesium aspartate, citrate, glutamate or glycinate are easier to absorb than the inorganic salts such as Magnesium oxide, sulfate, malate or taurate. It is best to speak with your physician and/or pharmacist and buy a form that works for you and that won't interact with your prescription medications.

If you take a form of magnesium that is too difficult to absorb or if you take too much, you run the risk of developing diarrhea. I have not experienced that problem because I found a form that my body is able to absorb and I follow the instructions on the label. I will be taking magnesium the rest of my life because it has made a huge difference in my health and well being.

8

Three Conditions Caused by a Magnesium Deficiency That may be Reversed by Increasing Magnesium Intake: Anxiety

Chronic magnesium deficiency can cause changes in biochemical pathways that increase your risk of developing an illness given enough time. It is therefore in your best interest to check and see if you have any of the symptoms that indicate magnesium deficiency. If you do have symptoms take action now to increase your intake of foods high in Magnesium and take a supplement if indicated. Following are three conditions that may have resulted from or have been made worse, because of a magnesium deficiency.

Anxiety

According to the Anxiety and Depression Association of America, anxiety is the most common mental disorder in the United States.It affects 40 million adults.

How do people cope with stress, fear, trauma and other disturbing

events in their lives?

In the past several years, globally and in the United States, we've experienced an unprecedented level of fires, floods, tornados, and heatwaves. We're living through the COVID pandemic and now the global MPX (Monkeypox) outbreak. Will it ever stop? If you turn on the TV and watch the news you hear about the latest mass shooting, you see videos of "smash and grab" robberies that are occurring in broad daylight in the local mall. Closer to home we suffer financial stress, relationship stress and other countless stress provoking events.

Stress and magnesium deficiency create a vicious cycle. In an experiment, adrenalin was given intravenously to participants. Results showed that adrenalin decreases magnesium, calcium, potassium and sodium. When you're burning adrenaline, you are burning magnesium which could result in a deficiency if you don't have a large enough reserve of magnesium to draw on. There are multiple major metabolic processes that are affected by adrenalin. These bursts of adrenalin cause all muscles to contract, they elevate the heart rate, constrict blood vessels which in turn elevates blood pressure. Magnesium is used up bringing these processes back into balance. In the experiment, IV adrenalin is stopped and it takes about 30 minutes for the body to recover. Potassium measurements indicate that potassium rises back to normal levels during that timeframe but magnesium takes much longer to reach normal levels. Over time, without taking in enough magnesium to replace what's been burned up, the body become deficient. The magnesium deficiency then triggers its own type of stress on the body resulting in feelings of anxiety and in severe cases, panic attacks.

As we learned from the experiments, when you have a stress reaction your body dumps out adrenaline in the "flight or fight response."

Magnesium is then dumped into your bloodstream to counteract the adrenalin response. If you suffer from chronic stress, your magnesium stores will eventually become depleted. If you are not aware of this vicious cycle, you may take medications for anxiety or depression when in reality, you need to address the deeper problem, which is a deficiency of magnesium. Any other medication is going to deal with the symptoms, but the root cause will not be addressed.

What is the first step towards resolving anxiety? Replace magnesium if you are deficient. Anxiety is a multifaceted condition and can have many triggering factors such as using too much caffeine, not getting enough sleep, working or living under stressful conditions. The list goes on and on. The treatment must address all the root causes including eating a good quality, whole foods diet, staying hydrated, practicing cognitive behavior therapy, getting more exercise, getting enough quality sleep, taking your medications as prescribed. This topic is greater than the scope of this guide, but you get the picture.

9

Depression

According to statistics published in 2020 by the National Institute of Mental Health, an estimated 14.8 million adults aged 18 and older experienced at least one major depressive episode. In other words, about 6% of adults in the United States were affected.

CDC statistics report that during the date range of August 2020 through February 2021, the percentage of adults with symptoms of anxiety or depressive disorder increased from 36.4% to 41.5%.

The COVID pandemic most likely contributed to this upward trend although the incidence of depression has been increasing from year to year and is caused by many factors. The following list will help you understand some of the causes of depression. If you are one of millions of people who suffer from depression, work with your physician to identify the root causes. Together with your physician, develop a plan that will treat your depression.

Risk Factors that Contribute to Depression

Physical Risk Factors

- Inherited genetic make-up: There are multiple genes which are associated with depression but they must be triggered by lifestyle, trauma or other conditions
- Age: Teenagers are at higher risk of developing depression
- Gender: Women suffer depression three time more than men. The younger a woman starts menstruating, the higher her risk of developing depression
- Ethnic: Latinx and Black teenagers have higher risk than white teenagers
- Family history of depression increases the risk of developing depression
- History of head injury

Dietary Risk Factors

- Diet low in tryptophan. Tryptophan is a building block used by the body to produce serotonin.
- Diet low in omega-3 fats
- Folic acid deficiency
- Deficiency of vitamin B12, B6 and the B vitamins
- Elevated homocysteine levels in the blood. Homocysteine is an amino acid. Studies have shown that elevated levels are associated with stroke and heart attack. It has also been linked to depression

Environmental Risk Factors

- Lead
- Mercury

- Manganese
- Arsenic
- Bismuth
- Trimethyltin Chloride
- Other environmental toxins such as toluene, and organophosphates. These have not been fully studied yet, but there have been some reported cases. However, at this time more information is needed

Socioeconomic Risk Factors

- Sexual abuse
- Codependency
- Lower socioeconomic class
- Traumatic or other stressful events
- No social network

Lifestyle Habits

- Lack of exercise
- Disrupted circadian rhythms.
- Abuse of tobacco, alcohol, caffeine
- Substance abuse such as cocaine, heroin, fentanyl, others
- Not getting enough sunshine

Medical Conditions

- Stroke
- Heart disease

- Cancer
- Diabetes
- Premenstrual syndrome
- Insomnia
- Thyroid disease
- Adrenal gland disease

Medications

- Diuretics
- Some blood pressure medications
- Oral contraceptive pills
- Cortisone
- Nonsteroidal anti-inflammatory drugs
- Antacids and anti-ulcer drugs

This list is not all inclusive and as more studies are done, more information will surface. However, this list will help you identify risk factors in your life that can be addressed or reversed, thus decreasing your risk of suffering from depression. Once again, I encourage you to place a check mark next to each risk factor on this list that affects you. If you are experiencing depression, discuss the list with your physician and develop a medical plan together. Date the list and revisit it periodically to track your progress. Are you feeling better or should you schedule another visit with your physician?

Can magnesium improve depression?

There is an entire new branch of psychiatry that is evolving which looks to food as medicine. This is often referred to as "Nutritional Medicine." The rational is if poor diet choices can cause heart disease and clogged arteries or can affect your metabolism so that you develop Diabetes, then why can't it affect your mental health? Studies do show that vitamin and mineral deficiencies and poor diet choices can result in poor mental health.

A literature review of 25 different studies published in 2021 uncovered a strong association between a person's mood and B-complex vitamins, B6, and B-12, folate, magnesium, calcium, iron, zinc, and omega-3s. These findings underscore the importance of a whole food diet that is rich in vitamins and minerals, with special emphasis on dark green leafy vegetables and orange or red colored vegetables, whole grains and high-quality proteins.

A study published in 2014 found that people who had low levels of magnesium in their cerebral spinal fluid, also had lower levels of 5-hydroxyindoleacetic acid which is a metabolite of serotonin. What does this mean? What the study discovered is that low magnesium levels lead to low serotonin levels. Magnesium is used by the body to manufacture serotonin. If you are deficient in magnesium you will also be deficient in serotonin. [24]

As we have seen, depression has multiple causes including the nutritional deficiencies listed above. It would be too simplistic to say that magnesium will resolve depression for all people, but we do know that if you have a magnesium deficiency, taking a supplement and eating a high-quality whole foods diet is a strong first step towards reversing the condition.

10

Insomnia

Insomnia can be caused by many things. Some examples include low progesterone levels, alcohol use, drinking caffeinated drinks too late in the day, numerous medications cause insomnia as a side effect; anxiety may also contribute to sleep disturbances.

How does magnesium improve insomnia?

One mechanism of action is that magnesium binds to GABA receptors in the brain. This process makes it easier to relax and fall asleep. A study done with elderly participants found that magnesium improves sleep efficiency, and sleep time.

Another mechanism is described in a study that found magnesium deficiency decreases plasma melatonin in rats. Melatonin is a hormone that regulates night and day cycles and improves sleep. By treating magnesium deficiency, you can increase melatonin levels and this will help to relieve insomnia.

Take an inventory of your lifestyle. There are many actions you can take to improve your sleep.

Read the list below and address as many of the lifestyle triggers under your control that may be contributing to insomnia.

- Heavy caffeine use especially in the afternoon or evening
- Alcohol use
- Nicotine use
- Staying up too late on most days of the week. (Bedtime after 10 PM)
- Chronic stress
- Sleeping in a lighted room
- Variable bed times (Not having a routine bed time and wake up time)
- Too much screen time or working under bright lights in the hours before bedtime
- Sleeping in a room that is too hot
- Lack of exercise during the day
- Low melatonin levels. Please note that melatonin levels decrease with age.
- Some medications will cause insomnia.
- Eating too late at night or eating a heavy meal too late in the evening may contribute acid reflux which will disturb your sleep.
- Exercising too late in the evening may give you a "second wind" and keep you wakeful too late at night.
- Doing any activity that is too exciting late in the evening may keep you too alert to fall asleep.

Ensuring that you are eating a high quality, whole foods diet that is high in magnesium is the foundation to improving insomnia. If you are deficient as evidenced by a blood test or if you are experiencing many of the symptoms of magnesium deficiency then consider taking a magnesium supplement, soaking in an Epsom salt bath a couple of times a week, soaking your feet in an Epsom salt foot bath, or going to a magnesium float spa.

But in order to improve the quality of your sleep, you will need to address each of the lifestyle triggers that are present in your life. Below is a list of actions you can take starting today, that that will improve your sleep.

What can I do to improve my sleep?

1. Use Cooling Sleep Enhancing technology: Do an online search. Check the reviews. There are cooling blankets, cooling pads or mattresses for your bed or perhaps a room air conditioner is more your style. Choose a product that fits your budget and lifestyle.
2. Red Lens Glasses are worn while working on your computer, using your phone or watching TV in the evening before bedtime. Wear them 1-2 hours before bed and upon waking throughout the night. They cut out the blue light emitted from your screen. This will help keep your circadian rhythms intact which in turn keeps your melatonin levels in balance. If you are interested in learning more about red lens glasses, start your online search at https://truedark.com/product/twilights-classic/. Your search engine will send you other similar products. Find one that fits your budget. The alternative is to eliminate screen time the hour or two before bedtime. Caution, don't wear red lens glasses during the day as they may make you wakeful during the night. These are meant to be worn in the evening and at night.

3. Blue light blocking and amber colored glasses: Blue light blocking and amber colored glasses can be used during the day to reduce blue light stress on your eyes.
4. Binaural Beats: Some people find listening to binaural beats just before bedtime is soothing and helps them fall asleep. Binarual beats in the delta (1 to 4 Hz range have been associated with deep sleep and relaxation. Binaural beats in the theta (5 to 8 Hz) range are linked to REM sleep, reduced anxiety, and relaxation, as well as meditative and creative states Search YouTube to try it out.
5. Weighted Blanket: Weighted blankets have shown in research to having a calming effect on the body. They are used for sleep, anxiety, stress, sensory issues, and restless leg syndrome. You may find this helpful. Blankets come in different weights.
6. Caffeine: Stop using caffeine altogether or at minimum, stop using it in the afternoon. Experiment. Will a cup of coffee after 4 PM keep you awake at night? Heavy caffeine use in the afternoon or evening may be disrupting your sleep cycle.
7. Alcohol use: Avoid drinking alcohol in the evening and at night as it is a sleep disrupter. As liver enzymes metabolize the alcohol during the night, the blood alcohol level decreases, and this causes sleep disturbances by disrupting the normal phases of sleep that our bodies transition through each night. Alcohol can disrupt your transitions from deep sleep to REM sleep which causes you to wake up several times. Initially alcohol may make you feel sleepy, but as the body breaks it down, alcohol becomes very activating.
8. Nicotine use: Stop using nicotine if you want to improve your insomnia problem. Nicotine disrupts sleep and may increase your risk of sleep apnea. Nicotine is a stimulant. It will keep you alert but it may also cause you anxiety.
9. Go to bed at the same time each night. The hours before midnight will give you the most rest. If possible, begin your sleep routine

at 9:30 and plan to be in bed by at least 10 PM each night. Wake up at the same time each morning. Try and get some exposure to the sun as early as possible. This will help reset your circadian rhythms.

10. Stress: Eliminate stress. This is easier said than done. If your job is stressful, start looking for another job. At one time I worked in an operating room where two surgeons worked who regularly yelled at the nurses. We walked on eggshells around them. It was stressful just waiting for the verbal abuse. I soon realized that I wasn't getting paid enough to suffer the abuse or to see my coworkers suffer through it. It took a little time but I found another nursing position and I was able to remove that stress from my life. I have also had to cut out negative, stress-provoking people from my circle of friends. There are lots of things that are stress provoking that we have no control over. However, there are some things that we can chose to change. Take a look at your life. Are there things or people you can remove from your life that will decrease your stress?

11. Sleeping in a darkened room. I live in an apartment complex that is well lighted at night. I've purchased blackout blinds to cut out the lights that are left on all night for our safety. Check your budget, what can you afford? When I was first experimenting with sleeping in a dark room, I went to Staples and purchased a roll of white paper and taped it on my bedroom windows. It worked and I did notice an improvement in my sleep. Do whatever works best for you and your budget.

12. Exercise: If you want to improve your sleep, start exercising. It can be as simple as taking a walk around the block. If you're not in good physical shape now, start slow. Walk around the block or if that's too far, just walk to the mailbox. As you get stronger, go a little farther. Eventually you may find yourself walking two

to three miles or more. It's up to you. It's best to do this in the morning if possible because exposure to early morning sunshine will also help reset your circadian rhythm. A side benefit is that if you suffer from depression, sunshine will help with that as well. It is well worth mentioning here that if you are exercising too much and are not giving your body enough time to recover, that could be detrimental to your health. If you think this could be a problem for you, work with a trained professional to help you develop a balanced exercise plan.

13. Melatonin levels: Melatonin levels decrease with age. There are foods that naturally contain high levels of melatonin and they have been shown to raise melatonin levels in the blood. These foods include cherries, goji berries, eggs, milk, fish and nuts, but especially almonds and pistachios. Reducing screen time, sleeping in a darkened room, having a regular bedtime and other actions will also improve your melatonin levels. There is no recommended dietary allowance for melatonin. If you want to take a melatonin supplement, the typical recommended does is around 0.5 to 3 milligrams in the evening before bed. Once again work with your physician and speak to your pharmacist. Melatonin may interfere with your medications. Discuss taking melatonin with your doctor and pharmacist before you decide if you will use it or not.

14. Some medications will cause insomnia. Look up the side effects of medications you are taking and see if insomnia is a side effect. If you are taking medications that cause insomnia, work with your physician to discover if there is an alternative medication you can take. If not, perhaps you can take it at a different time of the day if it is a one time a day medication. Do not do this on your own. Work with your physician.

15. Eating too late at night or eating a heavy meal too late in the evening may contribute to acid reflux. It's best to eat your heaviest meals

at breakfast and lunch time and then eat a light dinner or skip it if you can. This will improve the quality of your sleep.
16. Exercising too late in the evening may give you a "second wind" and keep you wakeful too late at night. If you are not able to exercise in the morning, then try to exercise at least two hours or more before bedtime.
17. Bedtime Routine: Doing any activity that is too exciting late in the evening may keep you too alert to fall asleep. Instead, build a bedtime routine habit. By doing the same relaxing activities each night from 30-60 minutes before your desired bedtime, you will train your body that it's bedtime and to get ready to fall asleep. Some effective activities include listening to music, or practicing prayer or meditation. Prayer or meditation can be as easy as thinking back on the day and expressing gratitude. By practicing the attitude of gratitude, you can reduce anxiety. Thank God or your Higher Power for each good thing that is in your life today and you will find that your faith and attitude will improve. Deep breathing is another very effective practice as you lay in bed preparing to fall asleep. A very simple deep breathing exercise involves taking a long deep breath to the count of three. Then exhale slowly to the count of six. Do this three times before bed. You can slowly increase the length of the inhale and exhale. Try to slow down your exhale breath so that it is twice as long as your inhale breath. There are many ways to engage your parasympathetic nervous system but that topic is beyond the scope of this guide. You can discover more by googling parasympathetic nervous system.

11

Conclusion

Because magnesium is a cofactor in over 300 metabolic processes, symptoms of magnesium deficiency manifest in various ways. As you increase your intake of magnesium you will notice that your overall health and well being will improve. As I mentioned earlier, many of the conditions that are symptoms of magnesium deficiency are also caused by other factors. Magnesium is a simple, inexpensive first step towards overall good health. As you reverse your magnesium deficiency you will begin to notice an improvement in the symptoms you may be experiencing. Depression, anxiety and insomnia all share a root cause, magnesium deficiency. There is no one magic bullet as much as we wish there was. It will take time to reverse a deficiency. It may have taken years for you to become deficient and it may take several months to reverse. Don't give up. Magnesium is inexpensive and simple to take.

I wish you the best as you work towards improving your life and your health!

12

Resources

1. Magnesium deficiency. (n.d.-b). Retrieved September 11, 2022, from https://medlineplus.gov/ency/article/000315.htm
2. Rude RK. Magnesium. In: Coates PM, Betz JM, Blackman MR, Cragg GM, Levine M, Moss J, White JD, eds. Encyclopedia of Dietary Supplements. 2nd ed. New York, NY: Informa Healthcare; 2010:527-37.
3. Rude RK. Magnesium. In: Ross AC, Caballero B, Cousins RJ, Tucker KL, Ziegler TR, eds. Modern Nutrition in Health and Disease. 11th ed. Baltimore, Mass: Lippincott Williams & Wilkins; 2012:159-75.
4. Volpe SL. Magnesium. In: Erdman JW, Macdonald IA, Zeisel SH, eds. Present Knowledge in Nutrition. 10th ed. Ames, Iowa; John Wiley & Sons, 2012:459-74.
5. Magnesium deficiency. (n.d.). Symptoms, Causes, Treatment & Prevention | Healthdirect. Retrieved September 11, 2022, from https://www.healthdirect.gov.au/magnesium-deficiency
6. Gibson, RS. Principles of Nutritional Assessment, 2nd ed. New York, NY: Oxford University Press, 2005.

7. Witkowski M, Hubert J, Mazur A. Methods of assessment of magnesium status in humans: a systematic review. Magnesium Res 2011;24:163-80. [PubMed abstract]
8. Nedley, N. (2001). Depression: The Way Out. Nedley Pub.
9. Just a moment. . . (n.d.). Retrieved September 11, 2022, from https://www.sciencedirect.com/topics/medicine-and-dentistry/intracellular-calcium#:%7E:text=Intracellular%20calcium%20signaling%20regulates%20numerous,sequestration%20in%20the%20endoplasmic%20reticulum
10. BSc, A. A., PhD. (2022, April 12). 7 Signs and Symptoms of Magnesium Deficiency. Healthline. Retrieved September 11, 2022, from https://www.healthline.com/nutrition/magnesium-deficiency-symptoms#TOC_TITLE_HDR_2
11. FoodData Central. (n.d.). Retrieved September 11, 2022, from https://fdc.nal.usda.gov/fdc-app.html#/?component=0
12. Ranade VV, Somberg JC. Bioavailability and pharmacokinetics of magnesium after administration of magnesium salts to humans. Am J Ther 2001;8:345-57. [PubMed abstract]
13. Firoz M, Graber M. Bioavailability of US commercial magnesium preparations. Magnes Res 2001;14:257-62. [PubMed abstract]
14. Mühlbauer B, Schwenk M, Coram WM, Antonin KH, Etienne P, Bieck PR, Douglas FL. Magnesium-L-aspartate-HCl and magnesium-oxide: bioavailability in healthy volunteers. Eur J Clin Pharmacol 1991;40:437-8. [PubMed abstract]
15. Lindberg JS, Zobitz MM, Poindexter JR, Pak CY. Magnesium bioavailability from magnesium citrate and magnesium oxide. J Am Coll Nutr 1990;9:48-55. [PubMed abstract]
16. Walker AF, Marakis G, Christie S, Byng M. Mg citrate found more bioavailable than other Mg preparations in a randomized, double-blind study. Mag Res 2003;16:183-91. [PubMed abstract]
17. https://www.cdc.gov/nchs/data/nhsr/nhsr172.pdf

18. Facts & Statistics | Anxiety and Depression Association of America, ADAA. (n.d.). Retrieved September 11, 2022, from https://adaa.org/understanding-anxiety/facts-statistics
19. Seelig MS, "Mechanisms of interactions of stress, stress hormones and magnesium in consequences of magnesium deficiency on the enhancement of stress reactions; preventive and therapeutic implications: a review" J Am Coll Nutr, vol 13, no 5, pp429-446, 1994
20. Major Depression. (n.d.). National Institute of Mental Health (NIMH). Retrieved September 11, 2022, from https://www.nimh.nih.gov/health/statistics/major-depression
21. Vahratian, A. (2021, April 1). Symptoms of Anxiety or Depressive Disorder and Use of Mental Health. Centers for Disease Control and Prevention. Retrieved September 11, 2022, from https://www.cdc.gov/mmwr/volumes/70/wr/mm7013e2.htm
22. Madeghe, B. A. (2021, January 7). Nutritional Deficiencies and Maternal Depression: Associations and Interventions in Lower and Middle-Income Countries: a Systematic Review of Literature. SpringerLink. Retrieved September 11, 2022, from https://link.springer.com/article/10.1007/s40609-020-00199-9?error=cookies_not_supported&code=b9b3fd31-c6ca-442b-a5b5-ff6e5e0c220c
23. Kaur J et al., "Role of dietary factors in Psychiatry." Delhi Psychiatry J, vol. 17, no. 2, pp, 452-457, 2014
24. Abbasi b, Kimiagar M, Sadeghniiat K, et al., the effect of Magnesium supplementation on primary insomnia in elderly: A double-blind placebo-controlled clinical trial. J Res Med Sci. 2012 Dec; 17 (12): 1161-9. PMID: 23853635; PMCID: PMC3703169
25. Supakatisant C, Phupong V. Oral magnesium for relief in jpregnancy-induced leg cramps: a ramdomised controlled trial. Matern Child Nutr. 2015 Apr; 11(2): 139-45. doi: 10.1111/j.1740-8709.2012.00440.x. Epub 2012 Aug 22. PMID: 22909270; PMCID:

PMC6860204

26. Pacheco, D. (2022, August 22). Bedtime Routines for Adults. Sleep Foundation. Retrieved September 11, 2022, from https://www.sleepfoundation.org/sleep-hygiene/bedtime-routine-for-adults
27. Breus, M. (2022, September 10). Foods That Are High in Melatonin. The Sleep Doctor. Retrieved September 11, 2022, from https://thesleepdoctor.com/melatonin/foods-with-melatonin/
28. N.D., D. C. M. (2017, August 15). The Magnesium Miracle (Second Edition) (2nd ed.). Ballantine Books.
29. What Are Binaural Beats? (2021, April 15). WebMD. Retrieved September 11, 2022, from https://www.webmd.com/balance/what-are-binaural-beats

Printed in Great Britain
by Amazon